Lavender Essential Oil

Everything You Need To Know About This Wonderful Essential Oil

By Amy Joyson

I0417489

information is without contract or any type of guarantee assurance.

The trademarks that are used are without any consent, and the publication of the trademark is without permission or backing by the trademark owner. All trademarks and brands within this book are for clarifying purposes only and are the owned by the owners themselves, not affiliated with this document.

Disclaimer – Please read!

The information provided in this book is designed to provide helpful information on the subjects discussed. This book is not meant to be used, nor should it be used, to diagnose or treat any medical condition. For diagnosis or treatment of any medical problem, consult your own physician. The publisher and author are not responsible for any specific health or allergy needs that may require medical supervision and are not liable for any damages or negative consequences from any treatment, action, application or preparation, to any person reading or following the information in this book. References are provided for informational purposes only and do not constitute endorsement of any websites or other sources. Readers should be aware that the websites listed in this book may change.

"Aromatherapy is one of the most powerful yet safe healing modalities we have today. It should be considered much more in healing."

Terry Friedmann, M.D., 1993

Table Of Contents

Introduction

Welcome to the third book in this series on essential oils and their therapeutic application in aromatherapy. Those familiar with earlier books in this series will recall our introductory guide in which a number of different essential oils were discussed, each in rather concise detail. This book will delve quite a bit deeper into this analysis, this time placing the focus on one essential oil in particular – the humble yet versatile lavender oil.

Why, you might ask, with the remarkable abundance of essential oils to choose from, does lavender oil take position as the first in this series showcasing individual essential oils? The answer, as you read through this book, will quickly become apparent. However, to surmise, it is the combination of lavender oil's sheer versatility, along with its usability, safety and accessibility that makes it the perfect opener for the amateur aromatherapist (and thus, the best candidate for this volume). The very adaptability of lavender is profound – it can be used, for example, to treat stress and insomnia, fight bacterial and viral infections, and reduce pain and inflammation. Lavender is also one of the milder essential oils available for therapeutic use. Impressively, lavender can even be used as a key ingredient in cosmetic preparations and cleaning products! As postulated elsewhere throughout this series, lavender is – in the view of this author – truly queen when it comes to the world of essential oils.

The format of this book will be somewhat familiar to readers of previous guides in this series. In Chapter 1, we begin with an exploration of the history of lavender oil and its use, from ancient through to modern times. Also, included here will be a brief discussion of the therapeutic significance of lavender oil. Chapter 2 continues with a review of the key properties and chemical composition of lavender oil, including a detailed analysis of the factors that give lavender its various therapeutic attributes. Next, in Chapter 3, we will take a look at the typical extraction methods involved in obtaining lavender oil, including information on how to carry out this process at home. Chapter 4 will take an obligatory look at the safety requirements when working with lavender oil, while Chapter 5 will review some of the most common methods for applying essential oils generally. The remaining chapters (6 & 7) will explore some remedies and recipes for various ailments and conditions that may be treated using lavender oil, either alone or in a blend with other oils.

By the end of this book, you should hopefully have a firm grasp of the importance of lavender oil in the world of aromatherapy. More so than in previous books, we will cover in quite some detail the chemical properties of the oil, which can be of great assistance in gaining a practical understanding of how and why an essential oil has a particular therapeutic effect. Most importantly, this information nicely complements the 'what', 'how' and 'why' that form an essential part of one's aromatherapy education.

A History of Lavender Essential Oil

Lavender oil is derived from the steam distillation of the plant of the same name (typically, the *Lavandula angustifolia* species of the lavender genus), which is believed to be native to the Mediterranean region of Southern Europe and North Africa. Lavender is classified as a flowering herb and is a member of the mint family. It has enjoyed its position as a revered medicinal herb for some thousands of years, with evidence of popular use in nearly all major ancient Eurasian cultures. The Ancient Egyptians are known to have used lavender in the preparation of tinctures for use during the embalming process, while it was also found to be a key ingredient in the herb, spice and sawdust blend used to stuff mummies and aid with their preservation. Additionally, lavender was commonly used in Egypt in various cosmetic preparations. The Greeks also used lavender prolifically, however, their usage of the flower took on a more therapeutic bent than the Egyptians. There, the plant was used as a cure-all remedy for various psychosomatic conditions, from insomnia to insanity and beyond. The contemporary name for the plant is possibly derived from the Latin *lavare*, or 'to wash', which hints at the typical Roman usage of the flower. (Another potential etymological source comes from the Latin word *livindulo*, meaning 'livid or bluish'). Typically, lavender was used as an aromatic by the Romans to scent their baths, dwellings and clothing. Lavender was also used cosmetically by wealthy patricians throughout the Empire as a perfume and treatment for the skin and hair.

Whatever the true origin of the present day name of the plant, lavender has maintained a long association with cleanliness and purification, from ancient times through to the modern era. There is an abundance of evidence of a strong connection between domestic cleanliness and the usage of lavender as a purificant across cultures; here again, the etymological connection is clear. The word 'launder' is believed to have evolved from *lavendre,* which is the Old French word for the same term. Indeed, the use of lavender in instilling freshness in clothing and linens via special lavender infused washes was a common practice used by 'launderers' throughout history, with evidence of this practice existing across a number of different cultures. The appeal of lavender for use as a cleaning agent is certainly understandable; not only does the strong, yet pleasant scent of the flower mask any potentially offensive odors, but fabrics (and flesh) treated with lavender would have been noted to have kept cleaner for a longer period than those effects and persons treated without it. This would have seemed like a rather magical property in pre-modern times; however, we now know this attribute is due to the antimicrobial effect of lavender, which would work to kill bugs that generated nasty smells.

Yet, it is not merely the power of lavender to clean that has given this special plant such a revered place in history. The medicinal and healing properties of lavender have also long been observed and held in high esteem. We have already seen how the Ancient Greeks used lavender to treat various health related conditions. Interestingly, however, this tendency to use lavender for medicinal purposes is one that endured for centuries and was again a practice that permeated throughout various cultures. For example, grave robbers during the 17th century proliferation of the Bubonic Plague throughout France are rumoured to have maintained their good health (despite the extremely dangerous nature of their work) by washing in a powerful disinfectant known as 'Four Thieves Vinegar'. As one might expect, one of the principal ingredients in this prophylactic against one of history's deadliest diseases, was humble lavender. Though the narrative of this story likely has its foundations in folkloric mythology, there is colloquial evidence of lavender being used around this time to ward off the insidious 'Black Death'.

Lavender also has strong links to the modern foundation of the practice of aromatherapy. In fact, it is often viewed as the 'first oil' of the discipline, both in chronological and taxonomical terms. In the case of the former, it can be linked to a very particular moment in the history of aromatherapy, when Rene Gatefossé (a renowned French chemist) stumbled upon the remarkable healing properties of lavender oil. As with many great scientific discoveries throughout history, Gatefossé's encounter with lavender oil as an agent for healing was largely serendipitous. During an unrelated scientific experiment gone awry, the chemist received severe burns to his hands and arms. In a moment of desperation, he plunged his hands into the nearest available solution that could likely provide relief to his injuries – a large vat of lavender oil. Although Gatefossé is understood to have not been fully aware of the healing potential of lavender oil at the time, the remarkable qualities of the essence soon became apparent to him, as his injuries began to heal at an unexpectedly rapid rate. This experience soon saw Gatefossé begin a further scientific exploration of the therapeutic qualities of other essential oils. This eventually led the French chemist to become known as the 'father of aromatherapy', and one of the leading figures in driving a renewed interest in the remedial potential of essential oils in modern times.

However, it isn't simply because of its place in history that lavender is viewed with such pre-eminence in the world of aromatherapy. In taxonomical terms, there are many arguments for placing lavender oil at the top of the tree, especially when it comes to the oil's long list of remarkable therapeutic properties. As we have seen from the above historical accounts, lavender exhibits some very powerful antimicrobial qualities. Its prolific usage in cleaning and personal hygiene across various cultures is not coincidental; rather, the antibacterial effect of lavender that can help to kill bugs and germs is also effective in eliminating nasty odors. Additionally, its attribution as a key ingredient in the plague-fighting 'Four Thieves Vinegar' provides another hint at the oil's strong antimicrobial properties. While most modern users of lavender are unlikely to need to recruit lavender for use as a prophylactic against the Black Death, it nonetheless has a number of therapeutic applications for the remedy of a number of bacteria related complaints. Although its use as a prophylactic against disease in pre-modern times would perhaps have had more of a basis in mysticism than science, we know today that lavender can be relied upon as a powerful natural antiseptic. We will discuss all of these therapeutic attributes of lavender in more detail in later chapters.

As we can see from this brief introduction to lavender, perhaps no other oil has been more influential or remarkable in its consistent and common use among different cultures throughout history. Its range of uses has varied over time from disinfectant and deodorant, to antiseptic and relaxant, and many more. Today, lavender remains immensely popular, both for its unique fragrance and for its plethora of therapeutic qualities when used in aromatherapy treatments. With a broad understanding of the historical significance of lavender oil, we will take a detailed look in the following chapter at the properties that are responsible for bestowing such a mighty reputation upon this humble plant.

The Key 24 Properties Of Lavender Essential Oil

The chemical composition of lavender oil

Having briefly discussed the rich and storied background of lavender, this chapter will now take a slightly more detailed look at the oil's chemical composition and therapeutic properties. As mentioned above, lavender is famous for its sheer versatility, a fact owed to the plant's complex chemical make-up. *Lavandula angustifolia* (the most common species of lavender used in aromatherapy) is estimated to be comprised of over 200 distinct molecular components, all of which contribute to the various characteristics and therapeutic properties of the plant. The primary constituent of lavender oil is *linalool*, making up just over 50 percent of its total volume. This terpene alcohol compound is found in over 200 species of plants and flowers, and typically produces a floral, sweet scent. In lavender, this compound helps contribute to the flower's distinctive fragrance, and is believed to also lend the aromatic plant its characteristic calming properties. At least one clinical study carried out using rodents has found that linalool lowered stress related hormones and neurotransmitters in rats significantly after they had been exposed to stress inducing stimuli.

The next biggest compound by volume found in pure lavender oil is *linalyl acetate*, which makes up about 35 percent of the volume of lavender oil. This compound is an acetate ester (and precursor) of the abovementioned linalool, a slight chemical variation which further adds to the aromatic complexity of lavender oil. Linalyl acetate is also found in bergamot oil and is characterized by a distinct, fruity scent. Both linalool and linalyl acetate have a significant anti-inflammatory effect, and help lend lavender oil this particular quality. As a general rule,

14

higher quantities of linalyl acetate typically indicate a higher quality of lavender oil. This is due to the fact that higher quantities of this compound are typically produced when fresh lavender flowers have been used in this distillation process, and the distillation has occurred under optimal conditions (these 'optimal conditions' will be discussed further below).

Present in smaller concentrations in lavender oil, but equally important to its chemical composition, are α-pinene (found in rosemary and eucalyptus oils), limonene (the main odor constituent of citrus oils, and effective as a sedative and stress relief agent), 1,8-cineole (known commonly as 'eucalyptol' and as such, a key constituent of eucalyptus oil), camphor (which exhibits anti-inflammatory and anti-microbial properties), ocimene, 3-octanone, caryophyllene, terpinen-4-ol and lavendulyl acetate. All of the various components of lavender oil are believed to act synergistically, working together to provide this remarkable plant's distinct therapeutic profile.

The A to Z of lavender oil's therapeutic properties

One of the remarkable characteristics of lavender oil is the sheer variety of therapeutic applications it can have. Although it is commonly known to be effective in inducing feelings of relaxation, it also has many, many other potential applications. For example, lavender can be applied to treat wounds and burns, or reduce the inflammation from injury. We will now take a detailed look at the various potential applications of lavender, looking at some of the science behind each effect.

Antiseptic: Lavender may be applied as an *antiseptic*, as it exhibits antimicrobial properties capable of killing a number of different germs and bacteria which can lead to infection. An antiseptic is a solution which may be applied directly to the

15

skin to reduce the chances of sepsis or putrefaction occurring through bacterial infection. Antiseptics typically work by either inhibiting the growth of bacteria or by directly targeting and killing the germs; lavender acts in this latter way. An antiseptic is distinguished from a disinfectant in that the latter may be used to kill organisms found on inanimate objects.

Analgesic: Lavender is also effective as an *analgesic*, or painkiller. Many clinical trials have been conducted in attempts to measure the pain relief qualities exhibited by lavender, including for the treatment of perineal discomfort in pregnant women and as a partial substitute for conventional pain relief medicine. The analgesic effect of lavender is believed to be connected to the effect of linalool and linalyl acetate on the brain's limbic system.

Anticonvulsant: Lavender has shown some effectiveness as an *anticonvulsant,* reducing the occurrence and severity of seizures when used in conjunction with standard anticonvulsant medication. Though there is little in the way of a clinically researched explanation for why lavender acts in this way, it is thought to be connected to the plant's general effect on modulating an overstimulated nervous system. Again, this effect is connected to lavender's effect on the limbic system.

Antidepressant: Another interesting therapeutic quality of lavender is its potential for use as an *antidepressant* and *anti-anxiety* treatment. Clinical trials have shown the habitual oral administration of lavender oil has an effect similar to some benzodiazepines, a typical 'go-to' class of psychoactive drugs used for treating anxiety and depression. Again, this effect is understood to be connected to lavender's moderating influence on the body's nervous system.

Antifungal: Lavender is one of many essential oils that exhibits a powerful *antifungal* effect. This makes it effective at treating a range of fungal conditions, from athlete's foot to ringworm. Research carried out by scientists at the University of Coimbra in Portugal found that lavender oil is lethal to a range of different pathogenic fungi, including various species of dermatophytes and candida.

Anti-rheumatic: Thanks to the anti-inflammatory qualities of lavender oil, it may be applied as an *anti-rheumatic*. Anti-rheumatics, as the name suggests, may be used to treat rheumatological disease, such as arthritis or gout. This action works largely in conjunction with the broader anti-inflammatory properties of lavender oil (with inflammation being a characteristics symptom of rheumatological disease).

Anti-spasmodic: Lavender also shows promise as an *anti-spasmodic*, or muscle relaxant. It can be used to treat soft tissue complaints (such as back spasms), or spasms related to the digestive system, which may contribute to cramps or improper digestive function.

Anti-inflammatory: As intimated above, lavender oil exhibits a remarkable *anti-inflammatory* effect. This is typically attributed to the high concentration of linalool found in lavender oil (discussed earlier in this chapter), a compound which has been shown to significantly reduce inflammation in clinical settings.

Antiviral/Bactericide: Lavender is both a potent *antiviral* and *bactericide* agent, making it highly effective for the treatment of wounds and the prevention of infection (see *antiseptic* above). This makes the plant and its oil particularly effective when it comes to the treatment of superficial cuts and wounds.

Carminative: Lavender oil also exhibits positive effects when it comes to digestion. It has been shown to be an effect *carminative* agent, mitigating the production and expulsion of gas from the gastrointestinal tract. As such, it makes a good treatment for those suffering from flatulence.

Cholagogue: A *cholagogue* stimulates the flow of bile from the bile duct to the liver. Lavender has shown some positive effect in this area and may be used to encourage healthy function of the hepatic system. This can involve the treatment of related conditions, including hepatitis and jaundice. Subsequently, lavender is also a good agent for use during liver detoxification.

Cicatrisant: Lavender oil has also been shown to have a *cicatrisant* effect, as it can aid in the generation of scar tissue, speeding up the healing process for open wounds.

Cordial: Lavender oil can be used as one of the main ingredients in a *cordial*. A cordial is a tonic which is used to improve circulation and aid with healthy function of the heart. A cordial is taken orally, which is not a standard practice when it comes to the use of essential oils for aromatherapy treatments. Cordials containing essential oils should only be taken under the careful prescription and advice of a trained professional.

Cytophylactic: *Cytophylactic* agents encourage the regeneration of new skin cells. Lavender has been shown to exhibit some cytophylactic effect, making it a good dermal aging (wrinkle) and skin repair treatment.

Decongestant: Inhalation of lavender oil helps to loosen phlegm in the respiratory tract, making it a good *decongestant*. Its antiviral and antibacterial properties also help to fight colds and respiratory infections.

Deodorant: Thanks to a combination of its pleasant aroma and its antimicrobial and antibacterial properties, lavender oil can be effective in both masking and combatting the source of offensive smells as a *deodorant*.

Diuretic: Lavender also acts as an effective *diuretic*. This can make it effective as an aid for maintaining healthy function of the urinary tract, preventing urinary tract infections, and for promoting the natural detoxification of impurities.

Emmenagogue: As an *emmenagogue*, lavender stimulates uterine and pelvic area blood flow. This can improve some symptoms associated with irregular menstruation, and may also relieve cramping that can occur during a period. Please note, emmenagogues should generally be avoided by pregnant women as their use may stimulate unwanted early labor.

Hypotensive: Lavender has been shown to have some effect as a *hypotensive*, lowering blood pressure after administration. This corollary may be due to the stress relieving effects of the plant, as there is a proven link between high levels of stress and high blood pressure.

Nervine: Lavender also has a notable *nervine* effect, in that it works to calm an overstimulated nervous system. As such it is often indicated for treatment of patients presenting with anxiety, insomnia and restlessness.

Rubefacient: There is some evidence that lavender oil acts as a *rubefacient*, acting to redden the skin when applied topically due to its effect of causing dilation of the surface capillaries. This can have the effect of reducing local area pain, and encouraging healthy circulation.

Sedative: Connected to lavender's power to induce relaxation and calming is the oil's ability to act as a powerful natural *sedative*. This is typically associated with the effect of linalool on the limbic system, which helps to moderate the body's inherent stress response mechanism and induce feelings of calm and relaxation.

Sudorific: Lavender exhibits some *sudorific* properties, due to its ability to induce sweating in a patient. This can be useful for those seeking to carry out a detoxification.

Vulnerary: This term refers to the potential for an agent to heal wounds. Lavender exhibits excellent qualities as a *vulnerary*, due to its ability to treat infection and speed up the body's natural healing process.

Lavender Oil Extraction

Lavender oil, like many essential oils, can be easily purchased through a number of different distributors. However, there are a range of reasons why it may be preferable to attempt to extract your own essential oils at home. Fortunately, with the right equipment, the extraction of lavender oil is a relatively simple and straightforward process. Lavender oil is most often and best extracted via the steam distillation of the purple-hued flowering tops of the plant (although leaves and stems of the herb are sometimes included in the process). Although there are a number of other extraction techniques that may be used to obtain essential oils (such as solvent extraction, cold pressing and water distillation), steam distillation strikes a good balance between maximum quality and yield of essential oil. Extraction using this method will typically yield a concentration of a little less than 2 percent by volume of raw product. This means that for every kilogram of raw lavender flowers, around 20 grams of pure lavender oil can be obtained through a typical steam distillation. Given that lavender oil has a density of about .89 g/mL, this translates to just under 18mL of pure lavender oil per kilogram of raw product. Although this sounds like a rather insignificant amount in comparison to the amount of material used, it is important to bear in mind that most aromatherapy treatments only call for the use of a few drops of essential oil at a time. Given that there are approximately 40-50 drops per millilitre of lavender oil (depending on the species of lavender in question), this means that from each kilogram of steam distilled lavender flowers, we can obtain enough lavender oil for over 100 typical treatments!

With the proper equipment, it may be possible to carry out an extraction of lavender oil at home. There are a number of benefits behind this practice, including cost effectiveness, guarantee of purity and the sheer satisfaction of 'creating' your own essential oils. Despite the initial costs of setting up a home still (the main piece of equipment necessary for the extraction of lavender oil), the long term financial benefits of home distillation are significant. This is particularly true when one considers the expense of various essential oils when purchased through a third party vendor. While it is true that the most significant determining factor when it comes to the expense of an essential oil is based on the market price of the raw material in question, there is of course an added cost margin in terms of the extraction of the oil itself. Furthermore, when it comes to assessing the purity of an essential oil sourced through a third party, a great deal of trust in the vendor and its product is necessary. Some manufacturers of essential oils will use 'shortcuts' in an attempt to cut costs and increase output. Such tactics include the purity-compromising use of solvents to increase yield; increasing temperature and pressure during distillations above optimum levels to maximize output (which can lead to an inferior final product); the use of raw materials that are of questionable or inferior quality; and/or the re-distillation of spent raw material. Although there are many reputable essential oil vendors in the online marketplace, there are nonetheless a few bad apples that make claims of purity doubtful when purchasing these products. Ultimately, it can take just one negative experience to shake one's faith in the quality and provenance of essential oils produced by a third party. Perhaps the best way to completely eliminate these doubts is to begin extracting one's own essential oils at home!

Components of a still

With this in mind, we'll now take a look at the equipment and method needed to extract lavender oil in the home. The main piece of equipment required is what is known as a *still*. This is the system required to carry out a distillation, and can come in a number of different types. A still can vary in its expense, depending on the complexity of the components, and purity of the oil required. A prefabricated, purpose made still may, for example, cost anywhere between a few hundred and thousands of dollars. However, for most amateur enthusiasts, a model on the cheaper end of the scale should suffice. There are a number of online sources through which a simple still can be purchased. A good place to start your search is with a generic online shopping marketplace, such as eBay or Amazon. There are also a number of online resources dedicated to the art of essential oil extraction that can point you in the right direction for detailed information on obtaining and constructing your own still.

If you are feeling ambitious, and have just a little technical know-how, it is possible to build your own still, too! When putting together your own still at home, it is important to know the key components required for a still to function properly. The first of these is the *boiler*. This is comprised of both a heat source (typically a gas or electric burner) and a holding tank, which typically contains both the water needed to create steam, and the plant material from which the oil is to be extracted. The holding tank should contain a grate or upper tier (like that found in a vegetable steamer) in which the plant matter is contained. Alternatively, this arrangement may be comprised of two connected receptacles, one containing distilled water and the other the raw plant material. More expensive stills allow for the distillation process to be carried out below atmospheric pressure, which allows for the distillation to occur at lower temperatures. This can result in a higher quality of the final product, as lower temperatures mean less molecular adulteration of the volatile compounds that comprise the oil. In the case of lavender, this would see the oil contain higher levels of unadulterated linalyl acetate (which, as discussed earlier, breaks down into linalool at high temperatures). Pressurization is not an essential part of a still in this process, but may be desirable depending on the quality of the product sought by the distiller.

Other essential parts of the still include the *condenser*, through which the steam flows and is re-liquefied, and the *essencier* (or separator), which separates the plant essence from other elements. A condenser is normally comprised of a double-walled glass tube immersed in cold water, while the essencier is also made of glass and is shaped like a tube or pipette with a valve operated tap at the base. The hydrophobic nature of essential oils makes their separation from the other main constituent of the distillation – water-based *hydrosol* – a relatively straightforward process. As oil floats to the top of water due to having a lower density, essential oils generally form a layer at the top of a higher density hydrosol solution. This effect is accelerated by the hydrophobic relationship between essential oil and hydrosol. The latter may be retained as this contains some essence from the plant, and can have therapeutic applications (although generally with a less potent effect than a pure essential oil).

Generally, the best materials to use when constructing a still are stainless steel or glass as these can handle high temperatures required for distillation, are non-reactive and are easily cleaned of impurities between distillations (although copper and aluminium may be used, non-reactive materials are preferable). A homemade still will most likely be cheaper and more customizable compared to a prefabricated unit; however, it can take a bit more effort to put together, and is more likely to experience functional problems (depending on the skill with which the still is put together!). There are again a number of online resources that can be useful for designing and constructing your own still at home which can be found via a Google search. I would suggest doing ample research before deciding to put together and use your own still, and to weigh up whether a prefabricated or homemade still is right for you.

The distillation process

One should begin the distillation process by first preparing the raw materials. When it comes to lavender, it is generally only the flowering tops of the plant that are used in lavender oil extraction. For best results, the flowers should be cut cleanly from the stems to avoid any loss of oils through damage to the plant. Once the flowers have been prepared, they should then be packed relatively tightly into the top level of the holding tank. The lower basin of the holding tank is then filled with water and the upper tier of the tank and lid are closed firmly in place. Heat is then applied from the heat source and the distillation process begins. Shortly after the first noticeable amount of steam is produced and moves through the condenser, you will note the re-liquefied essential oil and hydrosol begin to collect in the essencier and separate, with the oil floating to the top. Because the ratio of oil to hydrosol is very small, it may take some time before the oil becomes visible at the top of the hydrosol. A close eye should be kept on the still during the whole length of the distillation with care being taken that the boiler does not run dry at any time during the process. If water levels are running low, simply add more distilled water to the boiler via the water inlet.

Once it is apparent that distillation is nearing completion (when the hydrosol begins to run clear), turn off the heat source. When the last of the steam has flowed through the condenser and liquid has stopped entering the essencier, the mixture should be left to stand for at least 15 minutes so that any oil that may be mixed with the hydrosol is allowed to separate and float to the top of the solution. Very carefully and slowly open the tap at the bottom of the essencier, collecting the hydrosol in a separate container. Again, this should be done very slowly, as any oil left to flow into the container with the hydrosol will be lost. If possible, a drip-by-drip process is best here. Keeping a keen eye on where the level of the oil is in the essencier, the tap should be closed quickly once the last drop of hydrosol has left the tube. The remaining essential oil may then be collected in a separate container. Essential oils are best kept in non-reactive, dark glass jars which reduce the chance of photochemical reaction occurring during storage.

Maximizing the purity and yield of a distillation

There are three main considerations when it comes to ensuring the maximum purity and yield of an essential oil via home-distillation. These include *quality, time* and *temperature*. Perhaps the most important factor when distilling essential oils at home is the quality of the raw materials used. For example, if one uses lavender flowers that have been freshly cut, harvested at an optimal time and have been grown without the use of pesticides or other contaminants, a more superior essential oil will be the end result. Meanwhile, a still of a higher grade material and construction can often lead to essential oils of a higher purity. More expensive stills which allow for distillation to occur in vacuum conditions (at lower than atmospheric pressure, and thus lower temperature) may also lead to a higher quality final product.

The remaining elements for consideration when it comes to essential oil purity and yield are all related to the metrics of the distillation itself. Time (that is, the length of the distillation process) and temperature (the heat applied to the boiler) both have an effect when it comes to the yield and quality of the final product. The variations on these metrics required for optimum results varies from oil to oil; lower temperatures, for example, can lead to a better yield in some cases, but may cause molecular damage to volatile compounds in others. In the case of lavender, the optimum time and temperature are low in relative terms (compared to materials with more 'locked in' oils, such as cedar wood). Generally, it is advisable to run temperatures as low as possible, while still generating a viable source of steam. Meanwhile, the time of distillation generally takes around two hours, however the distillation process may be halted when the hydrosol begins to run from cloudy to clear. Distillation should be carried out at least until this point to ensure maximum yield from the raw material used.

Safety

As a final but highly important note on steam distillation, it is incredibly important to remember that the distillation process can be rather volatile and should be therefore carried out with extreme care. One should ensure that all equipment is in good working order, and that all necessary precautions are taken when it comes to working with the high temperatures associated with steam distillation. Steam burns can be particularly severe, and one should take care that direct exposure to steam or the heat source in question is avoided. Furthermore, a still should never be left unattended during a distillation, as there is a risk of fire due to the use of a heat source.

Complete Safety With Lavender Essential Oil

Lavender is perhaps one of the safest and most benign oils when it comes to therapeutic application. It is renowned as having a certain mildness in its potency, which prevents it from being associated with some of the adverse reactions that may occur with the use of more volatile essential oils. However, despite its relative safety, lavender must nonetheless be treated with both care and respect when being used in the practice of aromatherapy.

As a general rule of thumb, all essential oils should be treated in the same careful measure and as though they have the potential to cause adverse reaction in a patient. Although lavender oil is one of the few essential oils that may (in a few special cases) be applied 'neat' (undiluted), this should never be done outside the prescription or supervision of a certified aromatherapy practitioner. As with all essential oils, lavender should always be diluted before being applied directly to the skin. Likewise, lavender oil (like all other essential oils) should not be ingested unless advised by a trained aromatherapist. Although lavender is one of a number of essential oils that may be consumed without toxic effect, the concentration of pure lavender oil may induce an adverse reaction in some patients.

Though, as mentioned above, the potential for an adverse reaction to lavender is relatively low, there are a few pathological responses to be aware of when carrying out a treatment with this particular oil. When taken orally, lavender may lead to digestive complaints including constipation or diarrhea, as well as headaches or dizziness. When applied to the skin, lavender may cause local or general irritation in some patients. However, perhaps the most serious contraindication which may be attributed to lavender oil is the incidence of what is known as *gynecomastia* in pre-pubescent boys.

Concentrated lavender oil is believed to have a disruptive effect on normal hormone levels when applied, in particular, to the skin of those in this demographic. The result is the pathological growth of breast tissue in subjects in this group. Relatedly, the use of lavender should generally be avoided in pregnant women as the effects of lavender on fetal development have not been sufficiently researched.

Before beginning any aromatherapy treatment, it is also important to carry out an assessment of the suitability of the patient for the said treatment. Notably, one should determine whether the candidate for treatment belongs to a 'high risk' demographic. Groups which should generally be excluded from aromatherapy treatment include the very elderly, the young and those experiencing acute illness. While certain types of aromatherapy treatment may be suitable in some cases importantly, aromatherapy should never be used as a substitute for medical care or treatment. Severe injury or illness requires medical attention by trained healthcare professionals, and should be sought immediately.

It is also important to consider the suitability of the other ingredients used in conjunction with lavender oil when carrying out an aromatherapy treatment. Though lavender itself may not present any serious potential for negative effects in a treatment, other components used in a blend containing lavender oil may result in an adverse reaction. When using third party blends, one should always try to be aware of the listed ingredients and any potential adverse reactions that may occur as a result of exposure to these other components.

General Guide to Applying Essential Oils

Those who are familiar with other books in this aromatherapy series will recall an earlier discussion of some of the techniques that may be used to apply essential oils for therapeutic purposes. Book number two, in particular, was entirely focussed on one of these potential application methods – massage. However, there are many other methods through which essential oils may be administered to a patient. This is particularly true of lavender oil, which, due to its milder nature means that it may be applied through practically the full range of treatment pathways. The following chapter will now explore these in some detail, providing guidelines and considerations for how to best deliver therapy vis-à-vis lavender oil.

Topical application

This is one of the most simple and direct methods for introducing an aromatherapy treatment. It requires very little technical skill; the applicant merely needs to determine *what* to apply to the body of the recipient, and *where* to apply the treatment for best results. When applied to the skin, the fine molecules of which essential oils are comprised permeate the dermis and enter the blood stream, circulating their therapeutic effect throughout the body. As a rule, topical application of essential oils should only be administered in diluted concentrations as the volatile compounds in some essential oils may cause an adverse reaction in some patients. However, due to the mild nature of lavender oil, it may be applied 'neat' in some special cases (although only under the direction of a trained aromatherapy professional). Some ways to topically apply essential oils include via self-application, massage, or diluted in bath water.

Massage

Massage is a great way to introduce essential oil treatment to an individual. It combines all of the advantages of topical application, with the added therapeutic benefits associated with massage itself. What's more, there are a number of very different massage techniques that can yield various benefits and treatment outcomes. For example, there is the basic 'Swedish' massage, the meditative 'raindrop technique' massage, as well as a number of other types that have a specific treatment focus (such as 'lymphatic drainage massage', for example). Massage can be a great way to induce relaxation, lower blood pressure, and treat muscle soreness, and can be used to complement the treatment aims of aromatherapy itself. Further to the topic of safety covered in the previous chapter, care should be taken to avoid massage treatment in patients who are experiencing acute illness (including those with fever), have open wounds or communicable disease, or tumours. Extreme care should also be taken when practicing massage with children and the elderly. If in doubt as to whether massage treatment will be appropriate for a given patient, seek the advice of a physician.

Those interested in a more in depth exploration of the used of massage in aromatherapy should consult the second book in this series, which is devoted to a thorough investigation of this art.

Inhalation

Inhalation can be a most suitable delivery method when it comes to aromatherapy treatment, for a number of reasons. First, it is one of the less invasive treatment options, as inhalation of the vapour of essential oils generally results in few complications for a patient. Second, inhalation takes advantage of the special aromatic qualities of essential oils, and the effect that they have on the body's limbic system. The limbic system is often referred to as the 'ancient' part of the brain. That is, it is one of the most primeval parts of the human anatomy, and is responsible for influencing much of basic human function as a result. Emotions, behavior and other rudimentary and atavistic psychosomatic processes are connected to and governed by the limbic system. The neural mechanism responsible for governing the brain's scent detection system (the olfactory system) is considered a part of the limbic system. Also included in the structure of the limbic system are the *hippocampus* (which plays a key role in the management of memories), the *nucleus accumbens* (responsible for reward, pleasure and addiction), and the *amygdala* (which controls the body's fear/stress response). Subsequently, the exposure of this system to aromatic essential oils can have a profound effect on these various primal functions.

Inhalation can be carried out in a few ways, but is typically split between *direct* and *indirect* inhalation methods. The former can involve, for example, the application of essential oils to a blank personal inhaler, or the addition of a few drops of oil to a steam basin. Indirect methods of inhalation focus on the general diffusion of essential oils and typically make use of some kind of whole room diffuser.

Ingestion

Perhaps the least common form of delivery of aromatherapy treatment, ingestion is nonetheless a suitable option in some cases. Some milder essential oils may be taken in this way when used in highly diluted concentrations. Lavender, for example, may be taken in specific cases as a circulation boosting cordial, or tonic. However, because of some of the risks of adverse reaction when it comes to orally administering essential oils (such as severe irritation of the digestive system), this type of treatment is best left to the remit of trained professionals. One should therefore, avoid taking or administering essential oils through this method as a general rule.

The Health benefits of Lavender Oil

As intimated above, lavender oil exhibits some remarkable qualities that can help to improve a number of different aspects of one's health, thanks to its broad range of remedial properties. This chapter will take a look at some of the general health benefits that lavender can provide. The following chapters will take a more detailed look at some ways in which the health benefits that lavender offers may be applied to treat various conditions related to the below areas.

Relaxation, Calm & Improved Sleep Patterns

Lavender is very commonly associated with its potential for inducing relaxation and relieving stress. As discussed in earlier chapters, this is largely thanks to the plant's effect on the central nervous and limbic systems. This effect can have significant ramifications when it comes to treating mild insomnia. One scientific study found that patients who inhaled lavender oil directly from a vial before bedtime enjoyed a greater amount of 'slow-wave' or deep sleep, compared to a control group who inhaled from a vial containing distilled water. Test subjects exposed to the lavender vial also reported feeling more alert and invigorated the following day compared to the control group. As discussed above, the sedative/calming effect of lavender is understood to be largely connected to the essence's influence on the brain's limbic system.

Healing

Although lavender is perhaps most commonly associated with the abovementioned power to induce calm and relaxation, it is arguably the aromatic's power of healing that is its most impressive therapeutic attribute. The reasoning behind such an assessment is the number of complementary properties exhibited by lavender when it comes to healing power, as well as the mild nature of the oil. To understand the sheer efficacy of lavender's restorative ability, we should take the example of a small cut and explore the ways in which lavender would work to heal it. First, lavender's analgesic and anti-inflammatory effects both work to ease the pain of the small injury and reduce swelling and inflammation. Next, the antiviral and antimicrobial properties of lavender help prevent the wound from becoming infected, which also speeds up the healing process. Next, lavender's properties as a cicatrisant encourage the development of scar tissue, increasing the rate at which a wound is closed. Finally, the cytophylactic power of lavender encourages the regeneration of skin cells, which both speeds up the healing of the wound itself and encourages the return of normal skin quality once the wound is closed over. Importantly, it is not just simple cuts that lavender can be used to heal. Grazes, burns and acne can all benefit from an application of lavender.

Treatment of Anxiety & Depression

Another significant therapeutic benefit that lavender can provide is relief from anxiety and depression. Again, this effect is believed to be best evoked through the olfactory/limbic system and the power of scent; however related benefits may also be enjoyed when administered through other methods. As discussed earlier in this book, there is a lot of colloquial evidence of lavender being used historically to treat mood disorders (notably by the Ancient Greeks), and there is a reasonable amount of science that backs up these age old claims. As mentioned earlier in this book, lavender has been shown to have a similar effect to some benzodiazepines, a class of pharmaceutical used to treat anxiety.

Healthy digestive function

As a carminative agent, lavender can go some way towards regulating healthy digestive function by calming gastrointestinal activity. Additionally, its power as an anti-inflammatory can help reduce swelling of the gut, and can provide some relief when it comes to digestive complaints such as colitis and irritable bowel syndrome. Additionally, high cortisol levels (typically influenced by stress inducing stimuli) can have a significant adverse psychosomatic effect on the body's gastrointestinal system. Lavender's demonstrated ability to moderate stress levels can therefore have a significant, if indirect effect on stomach complaints related to stress.

Improved circulation

As discussed earlier, lavender is both a hypertensive and a rubefacient. This highlights the effect of the oil on circulatory function, as the former encourages moderated blood pressure, while the latter promotes circulation in blood vessels close to the surface of the skin. When combined in a blend with other circulation boosting essential oils, such as ginger and juniper, lavender can act as a powerful agent for encouraging good circulatory health.

Detoxification

Lavender is one of a number of essential oils that can be used to help detoxify the body of impurities, and leave one feeling more refreshed and rejuvenated as a result. The oil's effect as a sudorific (which helps to encourage sweating, discussed above) can help purge the body of harmful toxins via the sweat glands, while its action as a cholagogue encourages healthy liver function and hepatic circulation. Due to the liver's central role in naturally cleansing the body of toxins and impurities, lavender can act as a quiet hero when it comes to keeping one's body clean and pure from the inside out.

Pure Lavender Oil Remedies

As discussed so far throughout this book, lavender exhibits a wide range of remarkable therapeutic properties which serve to highlight the power and usefulness of this wonderful essential oil. Many arguments can and have been made that lavender is the only essential oil so versatile that it can form the entirety of an aromatherapist's emergency toolkit! The following chapter is devoted to an exploration of some of the different ways that lavender oil can be used in its own right to remedy or improve various health complaints and illnesses. Lavender is perhaps best used in isolation when one wishes to maintain a very simple treatment course, or when access to aromatherapy materials is limited. Each section in this chapter will highlight a particular treatment area, and discuss the various ways in which lavender may be applied to deliver the desired effect.

Stress relief

As mentioned earlier, lavender oil is very effective when it comes to lowering stress levels, thanks to high concentrations of linalyl acetate, and related compounds such as linalool. This makes lavender a potent stress relief agent when used in aromatherapy treatments, and makes for impressive results even when used independently of other complementary essential oils.

There are a number of ways to administer lavender oil to best enjoy its stress relieving properties. The best results, however, involve some form of inhalation and subsequent interaction with the limbic system (the significance of which has been discussed in earlier chapters). Therefore, one of the simplest ways to administer pure lavender oil for the purposes of relaxation is through direct inhalation. This involves either applying a few drops of pure lavender oil to a blank personal inhaler (which can be used on the go, before a stressful job interview, for example), or using a steam basin or room diffuser to similar effect. Alternatively, massage can itself act as a powerful stress reliever, and there are a number of different massage techniques that may be employed to this effect. One particularly effective massage method when it comes to its ability to focus the mind and reduce stress levels is known as the 'raindrop massage technique'. The spatial constraints of this guide prevent this method being discussed in great detail; however, feel free to consult the previous book in this series (dedicated exclusively to aromatherapy massage) for a more detailed guide on this particular treatment.

Antiseptic agent

Covered in quite some detail earlier in this book was the powerful potential of lavender oil when it comes to application as an antiseptic. The reasons for this are manifold, with the antiviral, antibacterial, anti-inflammatory and analgesic qualities of lavender all playing a key role in this action. Due to these special qualities, lavender can be applied to the skin to help curb infection and the onset of sepsis, while reducing pain and speeding the healing process.

In order to enjoy the therapeutic benefit that lavender oil can provide as an antiseptic agent, it is best combined with a soothing carrier (such as aloe vera) to create an antiseptic ointment. This treatment can be applied to various minor injuries, including cuts, grazes and burns.

Antifungal ointment

Lavender isn't just a powerful tool when it comes to preventing infection from injury, but is also highly effective when it comes to fighting existing infections, too. As mentioned earlier, clinical research studies have shown lavender to be a very powerful antifungal treatment, and highly effective in eliminating a range of fungal infections, including candida.

As with the use of lavender as an antiseptic treatment, a blend of several drops of the oil with a small amount of a suitable carrier oil. In this instance, coconut oil makes for a superior choice as a carrier as it exhibits excellent antifungal properties in its own right, and makes for a good combination with lavender.

Insomnia treatment

Lavender, with its relaxant, sedative and calming properties, is a good standalone treatment for those struggling to get a good night's sleep. As mentioned earlier, these attributes of lavender have been tested and proven during clinical trials, and may prove to be one of the simplest, least invasive methods for helping to guarantee a restful night.

When using pure lavender oil as a treatment for insomnia, it is best administered via the olfactory system to enjoy the best benefits. This can involve simply directly inhaling unadulterated lavender essence shortly before bedtime, either straight from a personal inhaler or via a room diffuser. Additionally, the oil can be blended with a carrier and massaged into the skin for a similar effect.

All-purpose anti-inflammatory

Lavender's anti-inflammatory effect is one of the oil's most potent attributes. Indeed, one of the best things about this quality is the fact that it can be used to treat a vast range of conditions which can have inflammation as a symptom. For example, minor cuts and bumps, sports injuries, and even the symptoms of arthritis can be successfully treated with lavender. To create such a treatment, simply combine a few drops of lavender with a carrier oil of your choice and massage into the target area.

Lavender Oil Blend Remedies/Recipes

With the above demonstration of the therapeutic power of lavender oil in mind, this chapter will now turn to an exploration of the various remedies and recipes (which include lavender as a primary ingredient) that can be used to treat a range of conditions. The following will provide both the recipes for crafting a suitable treatment blend for each condition, as well as delivery techniques and suggestions.

Stress relief blend

While the previous chapter discussed the potential for unadulterated lavender oil to be applied as a remedy for stress relief, there is a reasonable argument that such a treatment is best served by the use of a blend of complementary essential oils. Certainly, lavender is best used as the principal ingredient in this type of remedy; however, there are a range of other suitable oils that can be added to the mix for the purposes of enhancing relaxation and lowering stress levels. The following recipe offers one such suggested amalgamation, and can be administered in a variety of ways. The best methods of application, however, are those that also encourage relaxation and minimize stress, such as massage, inhalation combined with meditative exercises, or a calming, oil infused bath. Studies suggest that techniques which are focused around mindfulness can help to reduce stress levels in a patient, and blunt the response and even physical size of the amygdala (the brain's stress response center) over time.

Ingredients:
5 drops of Lavender Oil
3 drops of Roman Chamomile Oil
3 drops of Geranium Oil

15mL of carrier oil (if applying topically)

Method:
Combine ingredients in a dark glass jar. This blend can be used through massage (particularly of the upper body/neck), inhalation, or with a few drops added to a hot bath.

Sleepy time blend

Discussed in the previous chapter is lavender's power to induce calm and sedation. Although the oil is great by itself when it comes to its ability to ensure a restful night's sleep, this can be accentuated with the addition of complementary oils that also aid with relaxation. Roman chamomile is also renowned for its calming and relaxing properties, while frankincense can be useful for calming and focusing an overly active mind.

This blend can be mixed with a carrier of your choice and applied to the chest before bedtime, or administered without a carrier via an inhaler. As mentioned in the previous chapter, it can be a great idea to administer a sleep/relaxation remedy via a whole room diffuser before bedtime so that everyone in the near vicinity can benefit from the effect of the treatment.

Ingredients:
5 drops of Lavender Oil
3 drops of Roman Chamomile Oil
3 drops of Frankincense Oil

Method:
Add oils to a blank inhaler or room diffuser. Administer treatment from 30 minutes to an hour before bedtime.

Acne treatment blend

Severe acne is an incredibly unpleasant dermatological condition that can not only cause ugly and embarrassing blemishes, but may also leave residual scarring that remain with a sufferer for life. A specially blended remedy can not only help to clear acne, but reduce the occurrence of subsequent skin damage. Lavender plays a key role in the below recipe by reducing the inflammation associated with severe acne, while encouraging the regeneration of new skin cells. A good pairing with lavender in such a treatment is tea tree oil, which has a very powerful antimicrobial effect, while frankincense can also help to reduce scarring. A good carrier for use with an acne remedy is jojoba, which has excellent skin repairing properties in its own right.

Ingredients:
6 drops of Lavender Oil
3 drops of Tea Tree Oil
3 drops of Frankincense Oil
15mL of Jojoba

Method:
Combine ingredients in a dark glass jar and shake well to combine. Apply to the affected area after thoroughly cleaning face with a gentle cleanser. For best results, apply treatment nightly before bed.

Burns treatment blend

As discovered by the 'father of aromatherapy' during the early 20th century, lavender oil is incredibly well suited as a treatment for burns. Its anti-inflammatory effect is the main driver of lavender's ability to improve the condition of burns, while the analgesic effect of the oil helps to ease the pain of minor burns. These properties are well complemented with oregano oil, which also acts as a powerful analgesic, and chamomile, which can help to heal burns. These oils are best blended with a soothing carrier, such as aloe vera. This remedy can also be applied to skin affected by mild sunburn.

(Please note, this remedy should only be applied to minor burns or scalds. More severe burns should be referred immediately to a physician or emergency health care professional.)

Ingredients:
8 drops of Lavender Oil
4 drops of Oregano Oil
5 drops of Chamomile Oil
15mL of Aloe Vera

Method:
Combine ingredients in a dark glass jar and shake well to combine. Apply ointment liberally to the affected area.

Fever relief blend

Fever is a common accompaniment to a number of illness and can cause a great deal of discomfort for the sufferer. The sudorific properties of lavender that help to induce sweating can encourage a fever to break, while the sedative properties of lavender can encourage the crucial rest that the body needs when fighting a fever. This blend also makes use of the anti-febrile eucalyptus oil, as well as the strong analgesic properties of peppermint oil.

Ingredients:
6 drops of Lavender Oil
3 drops of Oregano Oil
4 drops of Eucalyptus Oil
15mL of Grapeseed Oil

Method:
Combine ingredients in a dark glass jar and shake well. Gently apply mixture to temples and upper body when fever occurs. Reapply every 12 hours until fever is broken.

Scar/blemish treatment blend

There are a number of different things which can lead to scarring of the skin during the course of a life. Acne experiences during the teenage and young adult years can leave residual scars and pockmarks for the rest of one's life; pregnancy can cause very visible stretch marks; and the general wear and tear of daily life can leave all manner of marks on the dermis for the long term. Lavender makes a good soothing base as a treatment for affected skin, with its cyophylactic properties encouraging skin repair and the growth of new cells. Meanwhile, geranium oil helps to regulate skin elasticity and tightness, while neroli can help to reduce fine lines and sagging in the skin, while generating new cell growth thanks to containing the active ingredient *citral*. The carrier, jojoba, is full of vitamins and nutrients which are great for improving general skin health.

Ingredients:
8 drops of Lavender Oil
6 drops of Geranium Oil
5 drops of Neroli Oil
15mL of Jojoba

Method:
Combine ingredients in dark glass jar. Apply a generous amount of ointment to the affected area, nightly.

Arthritis blend

Arthritis is an inflammatory disease that can result in extremely debilitating pain for the sufferer. The anti-inflammatory and analgesic properties of lavender can provide effective relief from the discomfort associated with rheumatological disorders such as arthritis. Meanwhile, the use of roman chamomile and black pepper oils instils a soothing pain relief and anti-inflammatory effect. Olive oil, as the suggested carrier oil in this blend has also been selected for its demonstrated anti-inflammatory properties. This blend can also be added to a hot bath (without the addition of the carrier oil).

Ingredients:
8 drops of Lavender Oil
4 drops of Black Pepper Oil
5 drops of Roman Chamomile Oil
15mL of Olive Oil

Method:
Add ingredients to a dark glass jar and shake well to combine thoroughly. Apply ointment liberally to the affected area a few times a day.

Eczema blend

Relief from persistent eczema is also one of the many potential therapeutic boons of lavender. This skin condition can be very difficult to treat effectively, but aromatherapy treatments have shown promise when it comes to alleviating its symptoms. This blend uses a combination of lavender, helichrysum and German chamomile work together to reduce inflammation, soothe itchy and irritated skin and reduce scarring. The jojoba carrier in this treatment is also great for the skin.

Ingredients:
5 drops of Lavender Oil
5 drops of Helichrysum Oil
5 drops of German Chamomile Oil
15mL Jojoba

Method:
Combine ingredients in a small dark glass jar and shake well. Apply ointment to the affected area twice daily, as needed.

Menstrual cramp blend

Lavender's action as an emmenagogue helps to encourage uterine blood flow, and can subsequently alleviate the pain and discomfort associated with menstrual cramps. This blend also makes use of clary sage and rose, which are both useful oils for treating issues related to women's health. Clinical trials have shown this particular combination of oils to be quite effective in reducing the discomfort, severity and occurrence of menstrual cramping.

Ingredients:
6 drops of Lavender Oil
4 drops of Clary Sage Oil
4 drops of Rose Oil
15mL of Grapeseed Oil

Method:
Mix ingredients together in dark glass jar. Massage gently into the abdomen when discomfort or cramping occurs. Apply every 4-6 hours as needed.

Sinusitis treatment blend

The pain of sinus congestion can be truly debilitating, and relief from the associated facial and cranial discomfort can thankfully be provided by aromatherapy treatment. Lavender's decongestant effect can really aid with clearing stuffed sinus passages, while the oil's antibacterial properties can help to fight infection in the area. This blend also calls on the cooling and analgesic power of peppermint, along with the antibacterial and disinfecting power of tea tree oil.

Ingredients:
5 drops of Lavender Oil
4 drops of Peppermint Oil
4 drops of Tea Tree Oil
Steam basin

Method:
Combine all ingredients together in a steam basin with hot water. Place head over basin with towel covering the head and the bowl to trap and direct steam. Take care when using this method to avoid steam burn from overexposure to direct steam.

Decongestant blend

Unlike the above sinusitis treatment, this blend may be used to treat congestion of the sinus passages as well as the lungs. Along with the decongestant and antibacterial powers of lavender, this blend relies on the similar and complementary properties of lemon and eucalyptus oils.

Ingredients:
5 drops of Lavender Oil
4 drops of Lemon Oil
4 drops of Eucalyptus Oil
15mL of Grapeseed Oil

Method:
Combine ingredients in a dark glass jar and mix thoroughly. Apply balm to the upper chest as needed, including before bedtime.

Antimicrobial blend

This blend can be applied to a range of different antimicrobial requirements, from use as an antiseptic ointment to apply to wounds, to a general sanitizing lotion. It makes use of lavender antibacterial and antiviral properties, as well as the complementary antimicrobial powers of clove bud, lemon, rosemary and cinnamon oils.

Ingredients:
5 drops of Lavender Oil
3 drops of Clove Bud Oil
4 drops of Lemon Oil
3 drops of Rosemary Oil
3 drops of Cinnamon Oil
10mL of Grapeseed Oil

Method:
Add ingredients to a small dark glass jar and mix thoroughly until combined. Apply to the affected area as needed.

Antifungal treatment blend

Fungal infections can be incredibly annoying, both in the discomfort they can cause to the sufferer, as well as their persistence. As discussed above, lavender exhibits a powerful and clinically proven antifungal effect, and thus makes a good basis for this blend. It is complemented here by the equally powerful tea tree oil, and clove bud essential oil. Coconut oil is used as the carrier, as it also exhibits powerful antifungal qualities and is high in vitamins and nutrients.

Ingredients:
7 drops of Lavender Oil
7 drops of Tea Tree Oil
3 drops of Clove Bud Oil
15mL of Coconut Oil

Method:
Combine ingredients in dark glass jar and mix thoroughly. Apply to affected area twice daily while symptoms of fungal infection are apparent, and continue for a week after signs of infection have cleared.

Exhaustion relief blend

Low energy levels leading to exhaustion can also be effectively treated with a blend containing lavender oil. This recipe calls on the calming power of lavender, combined with the focussing effect of frankincense and the invigorating effect of peppermint.

Ingredients:
10 drops of Lavender Oil
7 drops of Peppermint Oil
5 drops of Frankincense Oil

Method:

Add ingredients to a warm bath. Soak and relax in the bath for 20-30 minutes to enjoy the full effect of the treatment.

Jet lag blend

With international travel more commonplace than ever, jetlag is a condition that has been experienced by a growing number of people on a more and more regular basis. The calming power of lavender complements the rejuvenating effect of bergamot, while chamomile can help to reduce the occurrence of nervous irritability that can accompany jet lag. The below recipe suggests the use of a personal inhaler which can be prepared ahead of time and used during transit as a precautionary measure.

Ingredients:
4 drops of Lavender Oil
3 drops of Bergamot Oil
3 drops of German Chamomile Oil
Blank inhaler

Method:
Add essential oils to blank inhaler. Use inhaler as needed prior to and following the onset of jet lag symptoms.

Detox blend

There are a number of ways in which lavender oil can work as a good agent for detoxification. These have been discussed in more detail earlier, but will now be briefly recapped. First, lavender's sudorific properties allow the body to rid itself of impurities and toxins through the skin in the form of sweat. Secondly, as a cholagogue, lavender encourages healthy function of the bile duct and hepatic system. Finally, as a diuretic, lavender can work to rid the body of impurities through the renal system. These properties are complemented in the following blend with the equally powerfully detoxification agents, lemon and geranium oils. This remedy is best applied through massage to stimulate circulation and speed the detoxification process.

Ingredients:
6 drops of Lavender Oil
6 drops of Lemon Oil
6 drops of Geranium Oil
15mL of Grapeseed Oil

Method:
Add ingredients to a dark glass jar and shake well to combine. Massage a small amount of the blend into the skin twice daily for a week during the detoxification period.

Insecticide blend

During the hot summer months, insect repellent is a necessity. There are many commercially available insecticides which are highly effective, but also contain high concentrations of harmful chemicals, such as DEET. Fortunately, aromatherapy again comes to the rescue in this area, as there are many essential oils which can act as powerful insecticides. Lavender is one such oil, while eucalyptus and cedarwood are both also highly effective in this area.

Ingredients:
6 drops of Lavender Oil
5 drops of Eucalyptus Oil
5 drops of Cedarwood Oil
15mL of Grapeseed Oil

Method:
Combine ingredients in a dark glass jar. Apply ointment to exposed skin to prevent insect bites. Reapply every 1-2 hours.

Insect bite relief blend

If we are unable to keep insects from biting us, aromatherapy treatment may still be used to treat itchy or painful bug bites. The strong soothing and anti-inflammatory effects of lavender make it a good base for this blend, while oregano's strong analgesic effect can help with pain relief. Finally, peppermint can help to provide a cooling sensation which can help with itching and pain.

Ingredients:
7 drops of Lavender Oil
4 drops of Oregano Oil
3 drops of Peppermint Oil
15mL of Grapeseed Oil

Method:
Combine ingredients in a dark glass jar and shake well. Apply ointment to the affected area, as needed.

Anti-anxiety blend

Anxiety can be an incredibly overwhelming affliction and its treatment is not simply a desired course of action, but a necessity. Chronic and acute anxiety can have significant detrimental effects on one's health; indeed, the crippling symptoms of panic attacks are well known. Lavender's calming properties can have a significant effect in reducing anxiety levels. Additionally, frankincense can help greatly with focussing the mind, while clary sage oil is effective in calming the nervous system. Finally, Roman Chamomile is particularly effective when it comes to reducing anxiety levels. This blend is best prepared with an inhalation device and kept close at hand to deal with unexpected bouts of anxiety.

Ingredients:
5 drops of Lavender Oil
3 drops of Frankincense Oil
4 drops of Clary Sage Oil
4 drops of Roman Chamomile Oil
Blank inhaler

Method:
Add essential oils to blank inhaler. Use when feelings of anxiety begin to occur. Repeat as required.

Headache treatment blend

Headaches are possibly one of the most common health complaints around. Just about everyone knows the pain of headaches, which can be brought on by a wide range of associated health issues. This blend provides temporary relief from the pain of headaches, and is often a good alternative to reaching straight for a pharmaceutical treatment option. Lavender is a good lead in this blend due to its proven effect as an analgesic and relaxant, while peppermint boosts the pain relief qualities of the blend. Finally, Roman chamomile acts as an effective anti-inflammatory and also works as a sedative.

Ingredients:
5 drops of Lavender Oil
5 drops of Peppermint Oil
5 drops of Roman Chamomile Oil
Blank inhaler

Method:
Add ingredients to blank inhaler. Use at the onset of a headache, or as needed.

Upset stomach blend

An upset stomach can strike at any time, often when we least expect it. This remedy makes use of the anti-inflammatory and antispasmodic effect of lavender (which can assist with stomach cramps), along with its carminative effect (which can alleviate gas and bloating). Additionally, ginger oil is very powerful in terms of its ability to alleviate generic stomach complaints such as nausea and diarrhea, while peppermint exhibits and accentuates the effect of both lavender and ginger.

Ingredients:
5 drops of Lavender Oil
3 drops of Peppermint Oil
3 drops of Ginger Oil
15mL of Grapeseed Oil

Method:
Add ingredients in a dark glass jar and shake well to combine. Gently rub the lotion on to the stomach and reapply every 1-2 hours as needed.

Cold and Flu Remedy Blend

When the cold season strikes, we are all vulnerable to experiencing a bout of the sniffles. There are a lot of natural remedies out there when it comes to ways to fight and prevents colds and flus, and lavender is high on this list. The antibacterial and antiviral properties of lavender make it an effective tool for fighting colds and flus and other bugs. Additionally, the decongestant power of lavender can be useful in treating the symptoms of a cold. The antimicrobial qualities of this blend are further compounded by the inclusion of eucalyptus and lemon.

Ingredients:
8 drops of Lavender Oil
6 drops of Eucalyptus Oil
6 drops of Lemon Oil
Steam basin

Method:
Place ingredients, along with some very hot water, in steam basin. Place head over basin (with a towel over the back of the head) and inhale deeply. Continue for around 10 to 15 minutes.

Immunity boosting blend

Whether suffering from a generally poorly functioning immune system, or in an attempt to try and give a healthy immune system a boost, this blend can help to strengthen your body's natural defence against infection. Lavender and lemon both have great immune boosting properties and make a great treatment when added to a bath.

Ingredients:
5 drops of Lavender Oil
5 drops of Lemon Oil

Method:
Add ingredients to a warm bath. Soak in bath for at least 15 to 20 minutes to enjoy the full therapeutic effect of this treatment.

Respiratory function blend

Whether suffering from a chest infection or asthma, this remedy is a great treatment for healthy respiratory function. Lavender's decongestant and anti-inflammatory effects can help clear infect and reduce pulmonary swelling. Clary sage acts as an antispasmodic which can help with coughs and asthma, while eucalyptus acts as an expectorant. When treating respiratory complaints such as asthma, it is advisable to avoid directly inhaling essential oils, as this may lead to further irritation.

Ingredients:
6 drops of Lavender Oil
6 drops of Clary Sage Oil
4 drops of Eucalyptus Oil
15mL of Grapeseed Oil

Method:
Combine ingredients in a dark glass jar and mix thoroughly. Apply ointment to chest every 4 hours, as needed.

Ringworm treatment blend

Ringworm can be a bothersome fungal infection, resulting in an itchy, dry scalp and in some cases, hair loss. The condition can also affect other areas of the body, including the groin, hands and feet. The presence of ringworm can usually be identified by the distinct circular rash that accompanies an infection. Fortunately, ringworm can rather effectively be treated via aromatherapy and lavender, with its strong antifungal effect, makes a good basis for such a treatment. Additionally, the oil's soothing effect can help to alleviate the itchiness and irritation associated with ringworm infection. Aside from lavender, this blend makes use of the strong antifungal properties of tea tree oil, as well as the strong antiseptic effect of lemongrass oil.

Ingredients:
6 drops of Lavender Oil
3 drops of Tea Tree Oil
3 drops of Lemongrass Oil
10-15mL of Coconut Oil

Method:
Combine all ingredients in a small, dark glass jar. Mix thoroughly. Apply ointment to the affected area for at least a week after signs of infection have cleared. Keep the infected area clean and dry.

Sore muscle blend

This blend can be great for helping to relieve the aches and pains associated with sore muscles. Lavender's anti-inflammatory effect plays a key role here, while the muscle relaxant effect of Roman chamomile and the strong antispasmodic effect of thyme round out this blend.

Ingredients:
6 drops of Lavender Oil
5 drops of Roman Chamomile Oil
4 drops of Thyme Oil

Method:
Add ingredients to a warm bath. Soak for 15 to 20 minutes to enjoy the full therapeutic effect of the treatment.

Bruise treatment blend

Bruising, which is typically the result of soft tissue trauma, can be both painful and unsightly. This blend helps to heal bruises quickly after they have occurred. The lavender in this blend helps to both reduce pain and swelling from the bruise and restore the skin to normal health, while the helichrysum and geranium also assist in these areas.

Ingredients:
6 drops of Lavender Oil
4 drops of Geranium Oil
3 drops of Helichrysum Oil
15mL of Olive Oil

Method:
Combine ingredients in a dark glass jar and shake to mix. Apply ointment to affected area twice daily until there are no signs of bruising.

Lip balm blend

Dry and cracked lips are common and painful. This balm can help to restore natural moisture and return the lips and surrounding skin to good health. Lavender's restorative effect on the skin has been thoroughly discussed above and makes for an obvious lead in this remedy, while the jojoba, honey and beeswax have a nourishing effect on the skin.

Ingredients:
10 drops of Lavender Oil
4 tablespoons of Jojoba
1 teaspoon of Honey
1 tablespoon of Beeswax

Method:
Gently warm the lavender, jojoba and beeswax in a stainless steel pot over a low heat. Stir until the beeswax is melted and all ingredients are thoroughly combined. Remove pot from heat and sit atop a bowl containing ice water. Whisk in the honey, and once thoroughly mixed, transfer mixture to lip balm container. Leave in a cool, dry area to set for at least 3 hours. Apply balm to lips as needed.

Skin moisturizing blend

This remedy can provide great results when it comes to improving dry or irritated skin. Lavender has some excellent soothing and restorative effects on the skin, while rosewood exhibits some wonderful regenerative properties and jasmine is useful for treating irritation and toning skin. The carrier oils in this blend also have great moisturizing properties in their own right.

Ingredients:
10 drops of Lavender Oil
8 drops of Rosewood Oil
6 drops of Jasmine Oil
15mL of Avocado Oil
30mL of Jojoba

Method:
Combine ingredients in a dark glass jar and mix thoroughly. Apply lotion nightly to the desired area.

Sore throat blend

A symptom of a number of illnesses, a sore throat can be particularly unpleasant; however, this too can be treated effectively with aromatherapy. Lavender's analgesic effect helps with the pain of a sore throat, while its anti-inflammatory properties help to reduce swelling in the area. Lemon oil helps to soothe the throat, while the strong antimicrobial effect of eucalyptus helps to kill any germs in the area.

Ingredients:
4 drops of Lavender Oil
3 drops of Lemon Oil
1 drops of Eucalyptus Oil
Large glass of warm water

Method:
Add oils to glass of water and mix thoroughly. Gargle the solution, one mouthful at a time, for 30 seconds, and then spit the solution in to a sink. Continue until the solution is finished. *Please note, do not swallow this solution as essential oils may cause an adverse reaction if taken internally.*

Deodorant blend

Many commercially produced deodorants contain a wide array of metals and artificial chemicals that can have an unknown impact on our health. This blend offers a natural way to smell fresh, and relies on the classic usage of lavender as its backbone. Also included in this remedy is geranium, which has a nice complementary scent to lavender, and also exhibits a strong antibacterial effect.

Ingredients:
12 drops of Lavender Oil
8 drops of Geranium Oil
¼ cup of Baking Soda

Method:
Combine ingredients in a wide mouthed jar and stir with a spoon until mixed thoroughly. Take a small amount of the mixture in the hand and pat on to thoroughly dried armpits. For best results, use straight after showering.

Conclusion

As shown throughout this book, lavender is an incredibly important ingredient when it comes to the practice of aromatherapy. It offers so many different treatment angles with its wide range of therapeutic properties, and is second to none when it comes to its efficacy in delivering positive treatment outcomes in these areas using natural remedies. Lavender is also incredibly easy for the amateur aromatherapy enthusiast to work with, given the innocuous nature of the oil, its substitutability, and its sheer ubiquity and affordability. That lavender has held an important place throughout history is no mere coincidence. This multitude of factors highlights exactly why lavender has maintained its place of prominence as a key go-to ingredient for countless apothecaries across many centuries.

While this guide has championed lavender as one of the most important essential oils in the context of aromatherapy, there are in fact many, many more that exhibit equally remarkable properties. We hope that this book has encouraged you to think about the potential that the world of aromatherapy holds, given the impressive potential of this one humble ingredient among hundreds of natural therapeutic agents. Future guides in this series will explore the potential of other key essential oils, and hope to add to the encyclopaedic knowledge of aromatherapy available to the reader.

I hope you have enjoyed the third book in this aromatherapy and essential oils series and that it serves you well in your quest to master the art of aromatherapy in your home. I encourage you to keep an eye out for future books in this series and look forward to providing you with more useful guides that will help pique your interest in the exciting world of aromatherapy!

2 FREE eBooks for you!

Guys, thanks so much for reading my book. I truly hope it served as a great introduction to lavender essential oil. As a token of appreciation I have prepared two free ebooks for you. Here is a bit of information about them!

The 10 Most Important Essential Oils

In this book we delve deep into the uses and applications of the ten essential oils that I consider to be the most 'essential'. For each oil I explain the key health benefits, teach you the therapeutic applications and provide specific safety precaution. I include one of my most useful remedies for each of the oils as well. So you will receive a deep knowledge of ten essential oils and ten brilliant remedies for free! It is a 10k word eBook, the same length as this one!

When you receive this ebook you will also receive a couple of emails from me a week containing even more information about the essential oils! I will endeavour to give you at least 5 recipes or remedies per week and also provide you with some great information on the lesser known essential oils.

Simply click here to receive the ebooks!

Or type this link into a web browser: http://bit.ly/1EuHgyn

The Ultimate Guide To Vitamins

This is another wonderful 10k word ebook that has been made available to you through my publisher, Valerian Press. As a health conscious person you should be well aware of the uses and health benefits of each of the vitamins that should make up our diet. This book gives you an easy to understand, scientific explanation of the vitamin followed by the recommended daily dosage. It then highlights all the important health benefits of each vitamin. A list of the best sources of each vitamin is provided and you are also given some actionable next steps for each vitamin to make sure you are utilizing the information!

As well as receiving the free ebooks you will also be sent a weekly stream of free ebooks, again from my publishing company Valerian Press. You can expect to receive at least a new, free ebook each and every week. Sometimes you might receive a massive 10 free books in a week!

Simply click here to receive the ebooks!

Or type this link into a web browser: http://bit.ly/1EuHgyn

About The Author

Hey there! I'm Amy Joyson, a lifelong student of holistic and alternative medicine. My journey began as far back as I can remember, my mother, a practicing aromatherapist, taught me value of natural remedies as a youngster. I don't think I could imagine a life without the essential oils if I tried, they are just so important to me. I am passionate about sharing their value with as many people as possible, which led me to writing my books. If you have read any of my books I truly hope they have added value to your life and I thank you with all my heart for trusting in me.

Outside of being an author, I work as a personal trainer. Employing my deep knowledge of alternative treatments has enabled me to provide outstanding results for all of my clients!

In my spare time you will often find me lounging in my hammock reading the latest aromatherapy magazine or romantic fiction novel. I have a soft spot for true romance! I aim to meditate at least once a day, and practice yoga 5 times a week. My biggest hobby however is exploring the beautiful world that we live in. Next on my hit list is Iceland, there is something seriously alluring about that island.

You can find me here on Facebook:

https://www.facebook.com/pages/Amy-Joyson/435155886642915

You can find me here on Twitter:

https://twitter.com/Amy_Joyson

Valerian Press

At Valerian Press we have three key beliefs.

Providing outstanding value: We believe in enriching all of our customers' lives, doing everything we can to ensure the best experience.

Championing new talent: We believe in showcasing the worlds emerging talent by giving them the platform to grow.

Simplicity and efficiency: We understand how valuable your time is. Our products are stream-lined and consist only of what you want. You will find no fluff with us.

We hope you have enjoyed reading Amy's guide to Lavender Essential Oil

We would love to offer you a regular supply of our free and discounted books. We cover a huge range of non-fiction genres; diet and cookbooks, health and fitness, alternative and holistic medicine, spirituality and plenty more.

All you need to do is simply type this link into your web browser: http://bit.ly/18hmup4

Preview of "Essential Oils For Beginners"

I have included an example chapter of my first book here to give you a taste of the content. I really would recommend reading this book to gain a well-rounded understanding of the essential oils! Find it here:

http://www.amazon.com/dp/B00T12QLW4

"What are essential oils?

Simply put, essential oils are the concentrated essences (hence, the use of the term 'essential') of aromatic compounds. In Ancient China, these plant and flower essences were believed to constitute the 'soul' of the organism. These are often clear liquids and, contrary to the 'oil' in their name, often have a consistency more like that of water than of typical oils. From herbs, to flowers, to fruits, essential oils can be derived from many different organic sources. Around 400-500 essential oils are produced commercially, although there are many more types available. Essential oils are typically very complex, with single varieties often containing hundreds of individual aromatic compounds. As essential oils are derived from natural sources, they contain no harmful or synthetic chemicals which can have unknown detrimental effects on the body.

Essential oils are a key ingredient in many of today's consumer products, particularly in foodstuffs and cosmetics. They are also the subject around which the practice of aromatherapy is based. Essential oils hold great appeal to the individual due to their accessibility and usefulness. Not only can they be applied therapeutically, but also in foods, for household cleaning solutions, or simply for their distinctive aromatic properties. There are few tinctures which have such numerous practical applications, and are locked within the natural world that surrounds us, ready to be released.

How are essential oils obtained?

The process of extracting essential oils varies, largely depending upon the source material and available technologies. The oldest and perhaps simplest method of extracting essential oils is a process known as *enfleurage*. A relatively simple method, this involves crushing the product from which the oils are to be derived, and mixing the resulting powder or paste with a lipid (such as olive or vegetable oil). The oils from the source product permeate the lipids, and the essential oil infused mixture is then processed to be separated from the product residue. Though yielding a rather crude final result, this was a common method due to the lack of knowledge and expertise surrounding more complex extractions. The process for exploiting essential oils became more sophisticated over time. Archaeological evidence from the Middle East, such as pottery stills containing the residue of aromatic compounds, indicates that advanced extraction techniques were already being practiced in ancient times. Today, more sophisticated extraction methods mean that we can obtain highly pure and refined essential oils. The most pure essential oils are obtained through a process of steam distillation, whereby a solution is made from the source product, which is then heated, evaporating the essential oils. These are later collected through condensation after being cooled further along the system. The purity of essential oils is especially important when it comes to their therapeutic administration.

Another technique used for obtaining essential oils is the use of *solvents*. The use of chemical solvents is generally unfavorable amongst professional aromatherapists as it is the least natural way of extracting essential oils. The idea behind the method is that all the solvents used in the extraction are removed but occasionally light chemical traces will be left in the product. In this method the plant from which the essential oil is to be sourced is dissolved in a chemical solvent. The most common solvents used are; methylene chloride, hexane and benzene. These solvents have a lower boiling point than the essential oils and so are evaporated off, leaving behind the pure essential oil.

One of the most popular methods of obtaining essential oils is *steam distillation*. It is a simple procedure in which freshly harvested plants are suspended above a vat of boiling water. The steam that emerges from the water extracts the oil from the plant. The rising steam is captured and pushed through a tube before being cooled. As the steam condenses back into water, the essential oil (which doesn't mix with water) separates away.

Obtaining 'therapeutic grade' essential oils

In order to enjoy the therapeutic benefit of essential oils, it is vital that a product that is both high in purity and quality is used. However, essential oils that meet these requirements can be very expensive, due to the fact that a very high amount of organic matter is required to produce each milliliter of oil. In addition to this, it is much cheaper to extract the oils when sub-standard techniques are used. Typically, the extraction technique that results in the best quality oils requires both expensive distillation equipment and the expertise of a professional trained in its operation to perform the extraction. Sadly, the market for essential oils is severely lacking in regulation. Although, on the one hand this means that essential oils are readily obtainable, on the other, it makes certification of the quality of the product for sale difficult to verify for the individual. Therefore, as consumers of these important commodities, there are certain things we should look for, especially when shopping online for essential oils for therapeutic use:

- Is the information relating to the product thoroughly and adequately provided? E.g. Is the Latin name of the plant genus provided? Is the source of origin of the extract given?

- Does the product information state that the oils are 100% pure? Is there a suggestion that oils have been adulterated with other substances?

- When you receive the product, is it adequately and correctly labelled? Does the product smell as you would expect it to smell?

- Is the product significantly cheaper than normal market prices? If so, it is likely that the quality or purity of the product is compromised. (If it seems too good to be true, it usually is)

- Does the vendor seem legitimate? Do they appear to be knowledgeable about the product they are selling? Does the vendor seem trustworthy?

- Is the vendor you are purchasing the product from well-reviewed? If possible, try to find review of the company by third parties rather than relying on those that appear on their own website.

Although it can be difficult to guarantee that we are buying a legitimate product, particularly when shopping online, this can be true of any item – not just essential oils. It is important to carry out these basic precautions to protect ourselves as consumers, and to ensure that we are using a product of the highest quality. Remember; if you have reasons to suspect that the quality of an essential oil you have purchased is compromised *do not administer it therapeutically!*

How much should I be paying for essential oils?

As alluded to above, the comparative price of an essential oil is almost always reflective of its quality. However, there is no 'set price' for essential oils as such. All differ based on the expensiveness of the source material from which they are derived, and the volume of material required to produce one milliliter of essential oil. For example, take the case of essence of lemon. A large number of lemons are indeed required to produce one standard bottle of essence of lemon; however, because lemons are relatively inexpensive, it is normally one of the cheaper essential oils. A suggestion would be to compare the price of the oil you are looking to purchase to other reputable sites on the internet to make sure the price is in line.

How are essential oils administered?

Essential oils can be administered in a number of different ways. One of the most basic and effective methods (depending on the symptom being treated) is through topical application. This is not only true for treating topical conditions (e.g. such as skin irritation or bruising) but is also often a way to treat internal complaints (e.g. such as headaches or nausea). This method is connected to perhaps one of the most traditional ways to deliver therapeutic treatment in conjunction with massage therapy. When applied to the skin, essential oils are absorbed relatively quickly, as they are made up of very small molecules that are easily drawn into the dermis. This means that they are able to enter the bloodstream and take effect very quickly, compared to other therapeutic treatments.

A second way to administer essential oils is via either direct or indirect inhalation. In the case of the former, a personal inhaler is loaded with the oil(s) and their vapor is inhaled through the nose or mouth. For the latter, a vaporizer is typically employed, where the vapor of the oil(s) is diffused throughout a room. These methods are often best when treating an issue related to respiratory function, colds or flus, or sinus complaints. The final and perhaps least common method of administering essential oils is via ingestion. Though this technique can be suitable to obtain specific therapeutic results, it can be less safe than the above methods, particularly when not practiced or prescribed by a trained professional. Certain essential oils can damage the liver or kidneys when taken internally, or can interact with certain medications. Additionally, contraindications can occur when essential oils are processed through the digestive system. Always seek the advice of a trained professional if planning to administer essential oils via this method.

How do essential oils work?

From the three main ways that essential oils enter the body (dermally, or through inhalation or ingestion), the active ingredients interact with the body's systems in different ways. When taken through the skin, or via ingestion, the compounds from essential oils enter the blood stream acting much like a regular drug. They then circulate throughout the body and can have a localized effect on symptoms. Also when ingested, the ingredients from the oils are processed through the digestive system before being circulated through blood to the rest of the body.

When inhaled through the nose or mouth, essential oils interact with a number of different systems in the body. The olfactory system is responsible for controlling and effecting the sense of smell. As essential oils are highly aromatic, their interaction with the olfactory system can be an important part of their therapeutic application. Inhaled molecules also interact directly with the respiratory system, which can be a useful method of delivery when treating complaints associated with the respiratory tract and the lungs.

Finally, inhaled oils are believed to achieve some of their therapeutic outcomes by interacting with various receptors in the brain which constitute the limbic system. This system is thought to be responsible for a range of physiological responses, including heart rate, blood pressure, memory, breathing, and stress and hormone levels. This helps to explain why essential oils can have a profound array of effects on both human physiology and emotional well-being.

Why aren't essential oils backed as 'therapeutic drugs' by federal regulators?

One of the main issues surrounding universal acceptance of the 'therapeutic drug' status of essential oils relates to the dearth of clinical research evidence associated with them. However, this is not due to a lack of a link between essential oils and quantifiable therapeutic effect, but is primarily related to the fact that the number of clinical studies actually conducted in the area of essential oils has been limited. Many advocates of the therapeutic properties of essential oils claim that this is a result of two key factors. The first is due to the fact that drug companies have limited interest in sponsoring clinical trials in this area, due to a limited potential for profit. There is little to no money to be made from essential oils within the pharmaceutical industry, as they are natural products derived from natural sources, and therefore, are not patentable. Patents on drug design and manufacture are the number one source of revenue in the pharmaceutical industry.

Relatedly, the process for having drugs tested and certified by federal drug regulators is typically prohibitively expensive and depends upon the backing of the multibillion dollar pharmaceutical industry in some form. Thus, because backing by federal drug regulators *and* the pharmaceutical industry (who, because of the above may see the widespread therapeutic use of essential oils as contrary to their financial interests) are requisite for mainstream acceptance of therapeutic treatments, essential oils face a legitimacy problem. However, thanks to the limited clinical studies which *have* been conducted into essential oils thus far, we know that many of these products do in fact have clear antibacterial, antiviral and antifungal properties. This means that they can have a quantifiable effect on treating certain illnesses and conditions. Additionally, studies conducted on laboratory animals have shown that exposure to certain aromas under stressful conditions can improve behavioral and immune response. Finally, the amount of anecdotal evidence surrounding the positive therapeutic effects of essential oils is enormous. While not certifiable (as in the case of clinical evidence), this widespread popular backing nonetheless suggests that a significant multitude of people have used essential oils with great therapeutic results."

The book can be found here:

http://www.amazon.com/dp/B00T12QLW4

www.ingramcontent.com/pod-product-compliance
Lightning Source LLC
Chambersburg PA
CBHW072249310526
45795CB00011B/610